EYES ON SCREENS

How Screen Addiction
Shapes Visual Health in Kids

COPYRIGHT

TABLE OF CONTENTS

INTRODUCTION

Children are growing up in a digital age where displays, including those on computers, tablets, and cell phones, are everywhere. Their lives now wouldn't be the same without screens. Unquestionably, innovation has countless benefits but raises issues that must be carefully considered.

Screen addiction is a problem that extends well beyond our kids' electronic gadgets to their precious **vision**. The eyes of children—the portals to their souls—are at risk of possible vision problems due to endless scrolling, immense gaming, and the allure of social media.

Our top priority as educators, parents, and other caregivers is the welfare of our kids. We work hard to give them the best opportunity, to nurture and protect them, and to keep their health intact. Their vision is a crucial component of their well-being. It's not only about getting 20/20 vision; it's also about making sure their eyes stay healthy, bright, and unaffected by the allure of screens.

For anybody concerned about the welfare of children, this book, **"EYES ON SCREENS,"** is a thorough resource and a call to action.

We will begin a journey of comprehension, effort, and hope in the following pages. We'll explore the complex relationship that exists between screen addiction and how it affects kids' eyes, from the initial symptoms to any possible long-term effects. We'll look at the physical and behavioral signs of screen addiction that you might be missing. We'll present valuable tips for preventing screen addiction, protecting kids' eyesight, and helping them develop lifelong good vision habits.

This book offers concrete solutions in addition to spreading awareness. We will explore the digital terrain, highlighting the responsibilities of schools, parents, and caregivers in controlling screen usage. We'll also talk about how crucial it is to get expert advice when necessary to maintain our kids' vision at an optimal level.

Screens are here to stay in the digital age and present incredible educational, discovery, and relaxation opportunities. Instead of trying to remove our kids' access to screens, we want to help them develop positive and constructive relationships with technology. Together, let's set out on this adventure to safeguard our kids' most priceless gift—their Vision—against the effects of screen addiction.

CHAPTER ONE

Understanding Screen Addiction

In recent times, screens have become an essential part of our daily lives, especially for children. Kids are open to frequently accessing social media, games, and instructional information; therefore, computers, tablets, and smartphones have become their daily companions. Their adhesion to these gadgets has resulted in a propensity for extended and frequently compulsive usage, which is the root cause of screen addiction.

Defining Screen Addiction

Screen addiction is characterized by a compulsive urge for digital connection, frequently at the expense of other essential tasks. It goes beyond simply spending too much time in front of a screen. Other symptoms are the demonstration of irritability when not utilizing displays, neglecting obligations, and an obsession with digital entertainment.

Statistical Trends and Findings

There is scientific evidence of the fact that there is genuine screen addiction among children. A cross-sectional study among 400 randomly selected children aged 2 to 5 years in Chandigarh, North India, observed a high prevalence (Approximately 59.5% of children (mean age 3.5 ± 0.9 years)) of excessive screen time (Nimran et al., 2022). This is in line with similar studies conducted in the United States of America and other places in the World.

Screen Addiction is real, and we can no longer treat it as mere speculation. The evidence is ubiquitous - we can all find it around us.

CHAPTER TWO

How Excessive Screen Use Affects Vision

In this chapter, I delve into the connection between prolonged screen time and how it affects children's vision.

The Eye Structure

Let's pause to recognize the astounding complexity of the human eye before delving into the effects of extended screen time.

The human eye is a remarkable optical device comprising several components that function as a unit to allow us to see

our surroundings - the green plants, the beauty of sunset, our loved ones, etc.
The process of Vision is a true marvel of nature. Every object reflects light, and we see as a result of the amount of light that enters our eyes.

At first, light goes into the eye through the clear front part called the cornea. The cornea is like a dome and helps to bend the light so the eye can focus.

Some of the light goes through an opening called the pupil. The colored part of the eye called the iris, controls how much light goes through the pupil.

After that, the light goes through the lens, a clear part inside the eye. The lens and the cornea work together to focus the light onto the retina.

When the light reaches the retina, which is a sensitive layer at the back of the eye, special cells called photoreceptors change the light into electrical signals. These signals travel from the retina through the optic nerve to the brain. The brain then turns these signals into the images that you see.

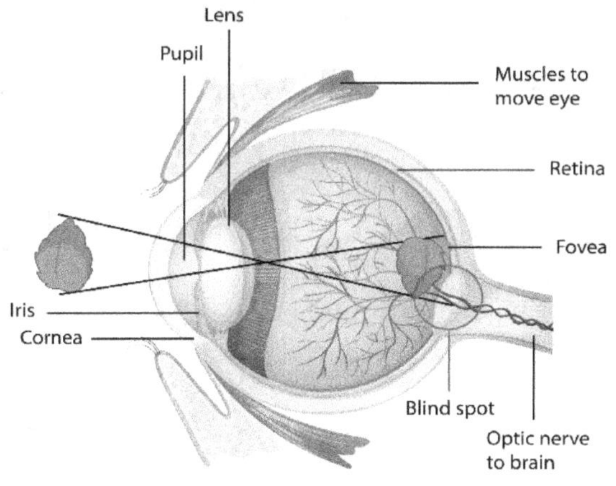

Image by brgfx on Freepik

The Impact of Prolonged Screen Time on Vision

The proliferation of screen usage, particularly among children, has raised concerns about how this constant exposure affects their Vision.

The following have so far been identified as some of the after-effects of long-term screen exposure:

A. The Rise of Myopia in Children

There is a strong link between children's screen usage and Myopia (Shortsightedness).

Myopia is a condition of the eye in which distant objects appear blurry while close things can be seen clearly.

It is commonly due to the elongation of the eyeball, resulting in light rays bent by the cornea and the lens falling in front of the retina instead of coming into sharp focus on it. Myopia also occurs if the refractive or light-bending power of the cornea is super strong causing light rays to come into focus in from of the retina.

Statistical trends reveal that the prevalence of myopia among children has been steadily increasing. The more time children spend indoors engaged with screens and the less time they spend outdoors, the higher their risk of developing myopia. Researchers believe that outdoor activities and exposure to natural light are protective factors for maintaining healthy eyes.

An article by the American Optometric Association noted that the lifestyle habits of children and teenagers today have vastly changed with technological advancements. It is noticed that the prevalence of myopia has been increasing for decades, and the increased level of near-visual stimulation from smartphones may pose an additional independent risk for Myopia (AOA, 2020).

Another research suggests that excessive screen time on digital devices may have adverse effects on children's eyesight. According to a study published in the journal PLOS One, school-aged children who spent seven hours or more per week using computers or playing mobile video games were found to have tripled their risk of developing myopia, commonly known as nearsightedness (CBS News, 2017).

Despite this, no study has yet proven that screens cause myopia, but there is a high association between screens and the development of myopia.

As an optometric practitioner, I have personally observed that many kids who have myopia have the habit of long-term continuous screen interaction. Some parents have confessed that these kids fixate on screens almost the whole day.

B. Digital Eye Strain

One of the primary issues stemming from excessive screen time is digital eye strain, also known as Computer Vision Syndrome.

Computer Vision Syndrome is a group of eye symptoms associated with prolonged computer or screen usage.

The symptoms of digital eye strain include:

- **Eye irritation**: Children often complain of discomfort and eye irritation after prolonged screen use. This may initiate the sensation of itchiness.
- **Headaches**: The strain on the eye muscles during screen time can lead to headaches. It is a common

complaint after extended screen time.

- **Blurry Vision**: Following extended screen exposure, children may experience temporary blurriness when they shift their gaze to objects in the distance. This may be due to over-straining the eyes; the eyes take some time to relax for clear distance vision.

- **Dry or Watery Eyes**: Reduced blinking while focusing on screens can lead to dry eyes due to the evaporation of tears, making the eye surface dry. Kids may complain of dryness, burning sensations, occasional itching, red eyes, and the feeling of foreign body in the eyes.

In some cases, dryness causes overproduction of tears instead, resulting in excessive tearing.

- **Squinting or Blinking**: Squinting or blinking excessively while looking at screens is another common physical sign of eye strain. These actions are attempts to alleviate discomfort and enhance sharp focus.
- **Sensitivity to Light**: Increased sensitivity to light is another symptom of digital eye strain. Children may find bright lights or sunlight particularly bothersome.
- **Double Vision**: Prolonged hours behind screens can cause

occasional and temporary double vision in kids.

C. Harmful Effects of Blue Light Emissions

Blue light, like other colors of visible light, is all around you. The sun emits blue light, as do fluorescent and incandescent light bulbs. Humans are exposed to more blue light than ever because of the widespread use of devices that rely on light-emitting diode (LED) technology.

Computer and laptop screens, flat-screen televisions, cell phones, and tablets all use LED technologies with high amounts of blue light.

Blue light is a high-energy visible (HEV) light with a short wavelength that emits significant energy. Long-term exposure to these harmful blue light emissions has detrimental effects on the eyes and may not necessarily be immediate, but later.

A publication by the American Optometric Association, categorically stated that visible blue light may be harmful to the human retina, as it can be absorbed by the retinal pigment epithelium (RPE) and specific photoreceptors, generating localized oxidative and thermal stress (AOA, n.d.).

D. Age and Vulnerability: The Impact on Developing Eyes

One primary concern is how developing eyes are susceptible to the effects of displays. Children's eyes are still developing, and too much screen time may interfere with this sensitive process. Because excessive screen usage at vital developmental stages may have long-term impacts on a child's vision, it is essential to consider this.

CHAPTER TREE

How to Recognize Signs of Screen Addiction in Kids

In our quest to safeguard our kids' eyesight and overall health from the dangers of excessive screen time, it's critical to identify the warning indicators of screen addiction. This chapter aims to provide parents, guardians, and educators with the knowledge necessary to recognize these symptoms and enable prompt intervention and support for our kids.

Behavioral Indicators of Screen Addiction

Recognizing screen addiction in children involves observing their behaviors and interactions with digital devices.

Some behavioral indicators to watch out for include:

- **Excessive Screen Time**: Children spend long, uninterrupted periods glued to their screens, often at the expense of other activities like social interaction, schoolwork, and physical play.
- **Preoccupation with Screens**: An obsession with devices, where children display irritability or distress when unable to access or use them.

- **Social Withdrawal**: Avoiding social interactions that do not favor solitary screen time leads to declining relationships and activities outside the digital realm.

- **Neglecting Responsibilities**: Failing to fulfill daily tasks, such as schoolwork or household chores, due to excessive screen use.

- **Preoccupation with Screens**: Children addicted to screens may constantly think about their next screen session. They may become obsessed with games, social media, or other online activities, leading to a preoccupation that interferes with daily life.

Decreased Academic Performance: Both screen addiction and eye strain can contribute to a decline in academic performance. Children may have difficulty focusing on their studies and struggle with reading or completing assignments.

- **Sleep Disturbances**: Children addicted to screens may experience sleep disturbances, such as difficulty falling asleep or waking up frequently at night. This happens due to blue light tricking the brain into believing it's daytime. When this happens, the body stops producing melatonin, a sleep hormone that helps the body relax and get ready for sleep.

The disruption of their sleep patterns can exacerbate eye strain and other symptoms.

- **Recognizing the Interplay**: It's important to note that screen addiction and eye strain often go hand in hand. A child addicted to screens is more likely to experience eye strain. The discomfort caused by eye strain may turn screens into a source of relief. This interplay complicates the recognition and management of these issues.

Creating an open dialogue with children about screen usage and its impact on their eyes is essential. Encouraging them to express their concerns and feelings regarding screen time fosters trust and aids in identifying potential issues and bringing about timely resolution.

CHAPTER FOUR

How to Mitigate Screen Addiction

This chapter will explore practical tactics and methods that can lessen screen addiction while protecting and maintaining kids' eyesight.

A.Setting Screen Time Guidelines

Establishing clear and consistent screen time guidelines is crucial in managing children's screen use. Creating a balance between screen time and other activities is essential for their well-being. The American Academy of Pediatrics recommends specific guidelines based on age, advocating for limited screen time and promoting healthy alternatives.

The AAP's guidelines allow some screen time for children younger than two (2). For this age group, parental involvement is essential.

They recommend the following for parents and caregivers:

- **Under 18 months**: Avoid screen time other than video chatting.
- **Age 18–24 months**: Find high-quality programming (if you introduce screen time), and watch or play together.

- **Age 2–5**: Limit screen use to one hour per day of high-quality programs.
- Create a family media plan with consistent rules and enforce them for older kids.

(Common Sense Media, 2022)

B. Creating Screen-Free Zones and Times

Establishing designated screen-free zones and times within the household is a practical strategy. Areas like bedrooms or dining tables could be designated screen-free zones, fostering an environment where screens are not the center of attention. Additionally, setting specific times, such as during meals or before bedtime, when screens are prohibited, encourages healthier habits.

C.Use of Parental Control Tools

Utilizing parental control tools and settings available on devices can aid in managing screen time. These tools allow parents to set time limits, restrict certain content, and monitor their child's screen usage. By using these controls, parents can ensure a safer and more balanced screen experience for their children.

D.Balanced Lifestyle and Diverse Activities

Promoting a balanced lifestyle that incorporates diverse activities beyond screens is critical to mitigating addiction. Encourage children to participate in hobbies, sports, reading, and social interactions. Providing alternative sources of entertainment and engagement can diminish their dependence on screens.

E. Encouraging Outdoor Activities

Outdoor activities play a vital role in countering screen addiction and preserving vision. Time spent outdoors offers a welcome break from screens and exposes children to natural light, which is essential for eye health. Sunlight exposure triggers the release of dopamine in the retina, which helps regulate eye growth and may protect against myopia.

F. Partnership with Schools

Collaboration with educational institutions is essential. Schools can support healthy vision habits by organizing outdoor activities, limiting screen time, and educating students about eye health.

CHAPTER FIVE

Ways to Alleviate Eye Strain

This chapter suggests practical ways to reduce eye strain and promote eye health and comfort when on screens.

A.Implementing the 20-20-20 Rule

The 20-20-20 Rule is a simple yet effective strategy to reduce eye strain. For every 20 minutes of screen time, encourage children to look at something 20 feet away for at least 20 seconds. This practice can alleviate eye strain by giving their eyes a momentary break from focusing on nearby screens.

B. Proper Screen Distance and Positioning

Encouraging children to maintain an appropriate distance from screens can significantly reduce eye strain. Ideally, screens should be positioned at an arm's length away, and the top should be at or slightly below eye level. Proper screen positioning helps minimize the stress on the eyes.

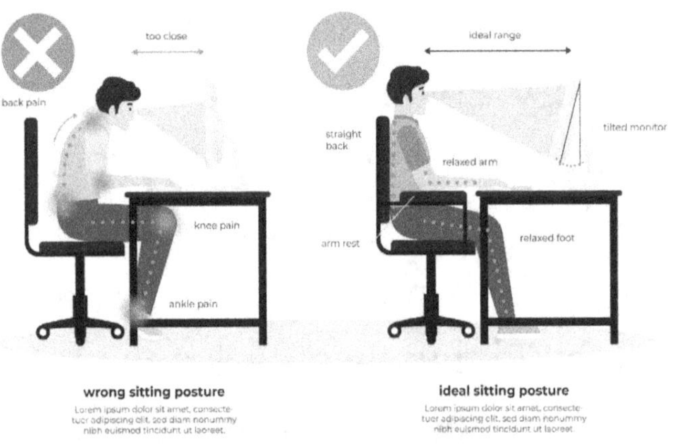

Image by Freepik

C.Anti-Blue Ray Glasses

Anti-blue light glasses are essential for children in this digital age. Anti-blue light glasses are special lenses that are made to block or filter blue light emitted, especially from digital screens. They have an anti-glare effect as well. These lenses protect the eyes from prolonged exposure to blue light, which might harm the retina, resulting in severe eye damage. Blue light glasses also reduce eyestrain and give good contrast and comfort when on screen.

D.Educating Children about Eye Health

Teach children about the importance of eye health. Explain the significance of breaks during screen time, the benefits of outdoor activities, and the role of good posture in maintaining healthy eyes.

E. Balanced Diet for Eye Health

A balanced diet rich in vitamins A, C, E, and zinc will help promote eye health.

Encourage children to eat foods that help improve vision, such as carrots, green vegetables, and fish.

CHAPTER SIX

Supervising and Regulating Screen Time: The Responsibilities of Parents, Schools, and Caregivers.

In our exploration of safeguarding children's vision in the digital age, we have examined the impact of screen addiction and excessive screen time, identified the signs of eye strain, and explored strategies to mitigate these effects.

This chapter delves into parents', caregivers', and educators' roles in managing screen time and promoting healthy vision habits.

Parental Roles in Managing Screen Time

A. Setting and Enforcing Screen Time Limits

Parents and caregivers are the primary gatekeepers of screen time for children. They must set clear and reasonable screen time limits based on the child's age and developmental stage. These limits should be consistently enforced to establish healthy screen habits.

B. Monitoring and Supervision

Supervision is crucial, especially for younger children. Parents should actively monitor the content their children access and the duration of screen time. This helps protect children from inappropriate content and ensures they follow the established screen time limits.

C.Leading by Example

Children learn by example. If parents are glued to their screens, it sends a conflicting message about screen time. Setting an example by demonstrating balanced screen use and engaging in alternative activities sends a powerful message to children.

D.Open Communication

Encouraging open communication about screen time and its effects is essential. Parents should talk to their children about the importance of balance, the signs of screen addiction, and the significance of eye health. A supportive and understanding approach fosters a healthy dialogue on the topic.

Educational Roles in Managing Screen Time

A. Establishing School Screen Time Policies

Educational institutions should have clear policies on screen time in schools. These policies can address the use of digital devices for educational purposes and should be designed to prevent excessive screen time during the school day.

B. Promoting Outdoor Play

Schools can play a vital role in promoting outdoor play in the curriculum. Incorporating physical education and encouraging breaks for outdoor activities can significantly contribute to reducing screen addiction and protecting children's vision.

C.Collaboration with Parents

Collaboration between schools and parents is essential in creating a balanced digital environment for children. Schools should actively communicate with parents about screen time policies, educational initiatives, and strategies for managing screen time at home.

D.Providing Educational Resources

Educational institutions can offer resources and information on screen time management and the importance of outdoor play. These resources can be distributed to parents and caregivers to increase awareness and understanding.

A Collaborative Effort

Safeguarding children's Vision in the digital age is a collaborative effort that involves parents, caregivers, educators, and the children themselves. It requires open communication, a unified approach, and a shared commitment to nurturing healthy screen habits.

CHAPTER SEVEN

Seeking Professional Help and Support

Professionals are trained personnel in their field of practice. Children are fragile in all respects, and having to do with their health, it is an emergency that should not be taken lightly. Therefore, it is expedient to seek professional service amidst the following:

A.Persistent Symptoms

Suppose a child exhibits persistent symptoms of eye strain, such as frequent headaches, blurry Vision, or discomfort, despite efforts to mitigate screen time and implement healthy vision habits. In that case, it's crucial to seek professional help. These symptoms may be indicative of underlying eye conditions.

B. Family History

A family history of eye diseases, such as Myopia - shortsightedness or other vision problems, increases children's risk.

Regular eye exams can help identify and treat these conditions quickly, reducing the risk of complications.

C. Impact on Academic Performance

If excessive screen time and eye strain begin to significantly affect a child's academic performance, then professional assistance is required. Struggling to see the board or read can lead to frustration, inattentiveness, and declining grades.

D.Signs of Screen Addiction

Recognizing the signs of screen addiction, such as withdrawal from social activities and excessive screen use, should prompt intervention. In cases where children cannot control their screen time despite efforts from parents, professional help may be required.

E.Changes in Behavior

Any significant changes in a child's behavior, such as increased irritability, difficulty sleeping, or a decline in physical activity, may indicate the need for professional evaluation. These changes can be signs of underlying health or vision issues.

The Role of Optometrists and Ophthalmologists

Regular eye exams by optometrists or ophthalmologists are essential for monitoring children's vision health. These professionals can identify vision issues early and recommend corrective and management measures.

An Optometrist (OD) - Doctor of Optometry is a primary eye care professional specializing in examining, diagnosing, and treating eye-related problems and visual disorders. Optometrists are trained to perform comprehensive eye exams to assess the eyes' overall health and prescribe and dispense corrective lenses (glasses and contact lenses) to improve vision.

An Ophthalmologist is a medical doctor (MD) or doctor of osteopathic medicine (DO) who specializes in the medical and surgical care of the eyes.

Prescription Glasses and Contact Lenses

If a child is diagnosed with Myopia, hyperopia, astigmatism, or other vision problems, prescription glasses or contact lenses may be prescribed. These corrective measures can significantly improve a child's vision and give comfort during screen time and other activities.

Treatment for Eye Conditions

In some cases, children may develop eye conditions that require treatment eg. dry eyes. Disorders like amblyopia (lazy eye), strabismus (crossed eyes), or more severe refractive errors may necessitate therapeutic or surgical interventions.

Mental Health Professionals

When it comes to dealing with addiction, professionals such as Counselors, Clinical Psychologists, Psychologists, and Psychiatrists are essential for helping individuals regain a sense of normalcy. These experts specialize in providing counseling and psychotherapy when needed.

These professionals conduct thorough assessments to understand the extent of screen addiction's impact on a child's mental health. They use standardized tools and interviews to identify any underlying mental health issues associated with or resulting from screen addiction.

After the assessment, mental health professionals create individualized treatment plans to address each child's needs and challenges. These plans may include a combination of individual therapy, family therapy, and participation in support groups.

In cases where screen addiction leads to severe mental health crises, mental health professionals offer immediate intervention and support. Collaborating with other healthcare professionals ensures the child's safety during crisis intervention.

Furthermore, mental health professionals collaborate with educators, pediatricians, and other relevant professionals to establish a holistic approach to addressing screen addiction. This collaborative effort ensures a comprehensive understanding of the child's environment, contributing to a coordinated intervention plan.

The Role of Support Groups
Support groups can be invaluable for children and their families dealing with screen addiction and vision issues. These groups offer emotional support,

share experiences, and guide on coping with challenges related to screen time and vision health.

The Importance of Timely Intervention

Timely intervention is crucial when dealing with screen addiction and vision problems. Early identification and treatment can prevent the worsening of conditions and long-term consequences.

ConclusionThe collaborative efforts of parents, caregivers, educators, and healthcare professionals strengthen our commitment to preserving our children's most precious gift—their Vision. Together, we navigate the path toward ensuring a healthy and thriving future for the eyes that behold the wonders of the World.

Thank You

REFERENCES

1. American Optometric Association. (2020). Children's myopia risk linked to smartphone use, study says. Retrieved from https://www.aoa.org/news/clinical-eye-care/health-and-wellness/children-device-use-and-myopia?sso=y

2. American Optometric Association. (n.d.). Blue light impact in children. Retrieved from https://infantsee.aoa.org/Affiliates/InfantSEE/Documents/Blue-Light-Impact-in-Children.pdf

3. CBS News. (2017, December 27). Too much screen time may be damaging children's eyesight.

CBS News. Retrieved from https://www.cbsnews.com/news/digital-devices-screen-time-damaging-childrens-eyes-vision/

4. Common Sense Media. (2022, March 11). How much screen time is OK for my kids? Retrieved from https://www.commonsensemedia.org/articles/how-much-screen-time-is-ok-for-my-kids#:~:text=They%20recommend%20the%20following%20for,day%20of%20high%2Dquality%20programs.

5. Kaur, N., Gupta, M., Malhi, P., & Grover, S. (2022). Prevalence of Screen Time Among Children Aged 2 to 5 Years in Chandigarh, a North Indian Union Territory.

Journal of Developmental & Behavioral Pediatrics, 43(1), e29-e38.

https://doi.org/10.1097/DBP.0000000000000964

www.ingramcontent.com/pod-product-compliance
Lightning Source LLC
Chambersburg PA
CBHW060842260726
48661CB00002B/556